LOW-OXALATE DIET COOKBOOK

AN EFFECTIVE DIET TO IMPROVE YOUR OVERALL HEALTH AND ENERGY LEVELS. WHOLESOME RECIPES TO TREAT INFLAMMATION, CHRONIC PAINS, AND KIDNEY STONES.

HALEY JOSEPH

CONTENTS

Introduction vii

INTRODUCTION TO THE LOW-OXALATE DIET

What are Oxalates?	3
What is a Low-Oxalate Diet?	7
Benefits of a Low-Oxalate Diet	9
Oxalate Diet Food List	17
High-Oxalate Foods to Avoid	19
Limit the Intake of Moderate-Oxalate Foods	23
Increase the Intake of Low-Oxalate Foods and Beverages	27

GETTING STARTED WITH THE LOW-OXALATE DIET

Tips to Follow and Mistakes to Avoid	33
Myths About Low-Oxalate Diet	41

RECIPES

Eggless Pancakes	49
Chive & Goat Cheese Soufflés	51
Belgian Waffles	53
Easy Tuna Pasta Salad	57
Cordon bleu Salad	59
Cherry Tomato Corn Salad	61
Tropical Turkey Salad	63
Beef Noodle Soup	65
Roasted Red Pepper and Potato Soup	67
Chicken and Rice Soup	69
Zucchini and Halloumi Bake	71
Spicy Ranch Cauliflower Crackers	75
Broccoli with Garlic and Chili	77
Baked Banana Chips	79
Green Beans, Ground Turkey and Rice	81

Grilled Pork Chops with Two-Melon Salsa	83
Pork Medallions with Grainy Mustard Sauce	85
Lamb Stew	87
Creamy Cherry Tomato & Summer Squash Pasta	89
Lemon Pepper Shrimp Scampi	93
Salmon with Creamy Dill Sauce	95
Creamy Chicken & Mushrooms	97
Fettuccine Alfredo with Chicken and Broccoli	99
Swiss Steak with Creamy Mashed Cauliflower	101
Creamy Pork with Sour Cream Sauce	105
Quick Roast Chicken & Root Vegetables	109
Rosemary-Lemon Lamb Chops with Potato and Fennel Latkes	113
Easy Paella	117
Lamb & Rice	121
Grilled Fennel-Cumin Lamb Chops	123
Strawberry Ice Cream	125
Peach Cobbler	127
Cranberry & Ruby Grapefruit Compote	131
Conclusion	133

© Copyright 2020 - All rights reserved.

The contents of this book may not be reproduced, duplicated or transmitted without direct written permission from the author.

Under no circumstances will any legal responsibility or blame be held against the publisher for any reparation, damages, or monetary loss due to the information herein, either directly or indirectly.

Legal Notice:

This book is copyright protected. This is only for personal use. You cannot amend, distribute, sell, use, quote or paraphrase any part or the content within this book without the consent of the author.

Disclaimer Notice:

Please note the information contained within this document is for educational and entertainment purposes only. Every attempt has been made to provide accurate, up to date and reliable complete information. No warranties of any kind are expressed or implied. Readers acknowledge that the author is not engaging in the rendering of legal, financial, medical or professional advice. The content of this book has been derived from various sources. Please consult a licensed professional before attempting any techniques outlined in this book.

By reading this document, the reader agrees that under no circumstances is the author responsible for any losses, direct or indirect, which are incurred as a result of the use of information contained within this document, including, but not limited to, — errors, omissions, or inaccuracies.

INTRODUCTION

Do you suffer from inflammation, bladder pain, chronic fatigue, or joint pain? Do you want to be rid of these problems? Do you want to improve your overall health without compromising your taste buds? Do you want to discover the secrets of healthy living? Are you tired of trying diets that promise results but fail to deliver? Do you want a diet that is easy to follow and sustainable in the long run? Do you want to do all this but don't know where to start? If you answered, "Yes," to all these questions, then this is the perfect book for you.

The busy and hectic lives we live, and all the stresses of modern living and poor diet, are the root causes of several health problems. To get through this, it is crucial to concentrate on your diet. Maintaining your physical health is the cornerstone of healthy living. Your diet not only influences your physical and mental wellbeing but the quality of your life too. If you are tired of feeling drained out of energy and are troubled by different ailments, shift your attention to the

Introduction

food you consume. The answer to all your problems is the low-oxalate diet.

Are you wondering what a low-oxalate diet means? It is a meal plan that is low in oxalates and helps heal your body from the inside. Many believe the low oxalate diet can reduce the symptoms of fibromyalgia, irritable bowel syndrome, bladder pain, kidney stones, and any other pain caused by oxalates in the body. This diet is ideal for anyone who suffers from kidney stones. It's not only curative but preventive too. The low-oxalate diet is believed to tackle inflammation, reduce the occurrence of kidney stones, flush out toxins from the body, restore the gut's health, and increase your energy levels. If you want all this, there is no time like the present to shift to a low-oxalate diet.

In this book, you will learn what oxalates mean, how oxalates are processed in the body, the meaning of a low-oxalate diet, and the many benefits it offers. You will also find a comprehensive low-oxalate diet food list and common myths about it. Once you understand this diet's basics, follow the simple tips and steps provided here to get started with this diet. In addition, you will discover several low-oxalate diet recipes. All of these recipes are not only incredibly easy to understand, but they are also simple to cook. You no longer have to compromise on your taste buds for the sake of health! Eat your way to a healthier you with the low-oxalate diet.

Learning about this diet is the first step toward a healthier body. So, are you eager to learn more about all this? If yes, let's get started by delving into the world of a low-oxalate diet!

INTRODUCTION TO THE LOW-OXALATE DIET

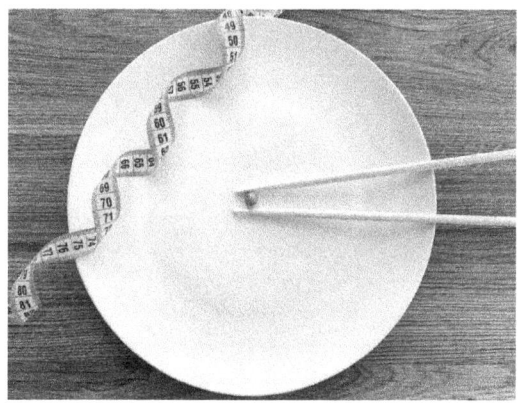

Making a dietary change might seem quite simple, but it is a major adjustment for your body. Most of us hardly pay any attention to our daily diets. This seems to be one of the leading causes for several health problems plaguing humanity. Before you decide to follow the low-oxalate diet, it is important to understand what it means.

WHAT ARE OXALATES?

You might have heard that avoiding oxalates is a straightforward means to prevent kidney stones. So, what are oxalates? Why is it important to understand how they work? Oxalates are known as anti-nutrients because they tend to bind themselves with important nutrients present in the body. This is a rudimentary explanation of oxalates, and their functioning is quite complicated. The level of oxalates present in food tends to vary. Many foods are rich in oxalates, while others contain trace amounts, but unless you understand what oxalates are and how your body processes them, you cannot make the most of a low-oxalate diet.

Oxalates are also known as oxalic acid and are natural compounds present in several plant-based foods. Due to their affinity to bind with other nutrients, they are known as anti-nutrients. So, why do plants need oxalates? The human body has its internal defense mechanism- the immune system. Similarly, even plants have a defense system, and the oxalates are a part of it. Oxalates or anti-nutrients offer natural protection to plants from predators such as insects, animals, and harmful pathogens.

In a way, without the presence of oxalates and other anti-nutrients, we might not have access to the wide variety of plant-foods today. Oxalates bind with different nutrients in the human body, but the helpful bacteria can break them down in the digestive system. However, in certain conditions, the accumulation of oxalates increases the stress on the kidneys and liver, preventing them from functioning optimally. Since kidneys and liver are the primary organs for detoxification, oxalate buildup results in various health problems such as kidney stones, chronic fatigue, digestive troubles, and so on. Most of these conditions are often caused due to the buildup of oxalates produced endogenously. Yes, oxalates are present in the food you consume and produced by your body.

How does the body produce oxalates? The amino acids, such as hydroxyproline present in the liver, are converted into oxalates. The red blood cells can synthesize oxalates from glyoxylate, and even vitamin C can be transformed into oxalates. Since oxalates can be synthesized from amino acids and proteins are made of amino acids, a diet rich in protein can also result in excess production of oxalates.

Now, let's look at how the human body processes oxalates. Whenever you consume food rich in oxalates, these molecules bind themselves with different minerals found in the digestive tract and, from there, they are eliminated from the body. Well, this might not necessarily be great news, especially for minerals, which are bound with oxalates (often calcium), but it is good for your body. It is safer for the body to eliminate oxalates instead of leaving them unbound. If the oxalates stay in their unbound state, they are eventually absorbed by your body and sent to the kidneys. In the kidneys, they are once again processed and eliminated as waste products.

If all these functions go on smoothly so there is nothing to worry about. But oxalates have an affinity to bind themselves with minerals, especially calcium is bad news for your kidneys. This is where things become a little complicated. Over a period, oxalates and calcium accumulate in kidneys and result in calcium oxalate kidney stones. This issue is further worsened if you don't drink enough fluids to eliminate oxalates from your body.

As mentioned earlier, different strains of gut bacteria help metabolize oxalates. High levels of helpful gut bacteria known as Oxalobacter formigenes promote the breakdown of oxalates. According to a study conducted by David W. Kaufman et al., the presence of Oxalobacter formigenes, a gram-negative bacterium, in high levels can reduce the risk of developing kidney stones. Research by R D Mittal et al. in 2005 showed that antibiotics can reduce the levels of this helpful bacterium. Without sufficient Oxalobacter Formigenes, oxalates tend to build up in the body.

The risk of kidney stones is closely associated with the health of your digestive tract. When the digestive system is running smoothly, oxalates are easily processed and eliminated through natural processes, but the presence of any digestive issues increases the risk of oxalate buildup. This is especially true for all those individuals with inflammatory bowel diseases and conditions. So, any alteration to have your digestive system functions becomes a risk factor for oxalates' buildup.

Another factor that comes into the picture is the levels of vitamin C in your body. High levels of vitamin C increase the buildup of oxalates. If your vitamin C intake exceeds 1000 mg per day, oxalate buildup increases, as demonstrated by the findings of John Knight et al. in 2017.

WHAT IS A LOW-OXALATE DIET?

As the name suggests, a low-oxalate diet reduces your oxalate intake. It takes into consideration the simple fact that oxalates are produced endogenously. By eliminating foods rich in oxalates and supplementing them with low-oxalate foods, you can reverse the harmful effects of oxalates. In 2014, research by Matthew D Sorensen found that consuming a diet rich in calcium, especially when you consume high oxalate foods, can reduce oxalate buildup. This works because oxalate and calcium bind together before reaching the kidneys and reduce kidney stone formation risk.

Unlike a traditional kidney stone diet that eliminates all forms of oxalate foods from your diet, the low-oxalate diet eliminates only high oxalate foods' consumption. Since most of the oxalate foods are rich in other nutrients and fiber, eliminating them is not a good idea. Instead, opt for a diet that stabilizes your intake and balances the volume of oxalates. While following a low oxalate diet, your daily intake of oxalates is around 40-50 mg per day.

BENEFITS OF A LOW-OXALATE DIET

Now that you know what oxalates mean and how the body processes them, let's look at the different benefits of a low-oxalate diet.

Say Goodbye to Weakness and Joint Problems

The human body has an internal maintenance system that regularly performs tissue maintenance and repair. From repairing damaged skin to strengthening weak joints or connective tissue, your body can do it all, but oxalates tend to interfere with regular tissue maintenance and repair. It can cause unstable and weak joints, easily damage the skin and its membranes, and can even result in persistent scarring. Your body's ability to recover from injuries and its healing ability reduce when oxalates start accumulating invulnerable tissues. It can also worsen or perpetuate any existing inflammatory conditions.

Apart from triggering inflammation and harming connective tissues, oxalates usually accumulate in joint spaces so that inflammation resulting from oxalate accumulation results in tightness of joints, joint degeneration, and general pain. As you know, oxalates tend to bind with calcium. Calcium is important for the maintenance of your bones and teeth. Calcium oxalate is formed when oxalate acid is combined with calcium in the body. This compound tends to accumulate in teeth, bones, osteoporosis, cracked teeth, Stenosis, and weak bones.

So, a low-oxalate diet helps reverse these conditions and improves calcium absorption to strengthen your bones and teeth. It also tackles inflammation and indirectly reduces the occurrence of pain caused due to inflammatory conditions.

Reduce the Risk of Kidney Stones

By consuming a diet rich in oxalates, the risk of kidney stones increases. Remember, oxalates are not only present in the food you eat, but your body produces them too. A common spot where oxalates start accumulating is the kidneys. The greater the absorption of oxalates from the digestive tract, the higher the chances are that it will reach the kidneys. This, in turn, increases the levels of urinary oxalates. The high levels of urinary calcium can increase the risk of calcium oxalate formation in the kidneys, resulting in kidney stones. The simplest way to reduce the risk of kidney stones is by following a low-oxalate diet.

Alleviate Immune System Reactions

Inflammation is your body's first line of defense against foreign invaders. In controlled amounts, inflammation is desirable because it protects your body, but when left unchecked, it can cause inflammatory illnesses and even trigger an autoimmune disorder. In an autoimmune dysfunction, the immune system starts attacking healthy cells. This adverse reaction is often triggered due to the presence of excess oxalates in the body. A common gland in which oxalates accumulate in the thyroid. Thyroid disorders and other inflammatory and autoimmune conditions can cause fatigue. Inflammation can also present itself as rashes and other skin troubles. By shifting to a low-oxalate diet, all of these conditions can be tackled. Inflammatory problems, such as rheumatoid arthritis, can also be controlled.

Better Gut Health

As you know, oxalates trigger inflammation. Certain oxalate micro crystals present in foods tend to have sharp and pointy edges. These glass-like structures harm the mucous membrane in different cells present in the digestive tract and system. Once the lining of the digestive tract is compromised, undigested food particles can enter the blood supply. These unsupervised food particles can trigger autoimmune disorders where the immune system mistakes them for pathogens. Oxalate crystals can slowly erode the digestive systems' inner linings. So they not only trigger digestive troubles such as the leaky gut, irritable bowel syndrome, diarrhea, constipation, and gastroenteritis, but they also can aggravate existing digestive problems.

Tackle Irritation and Dysfunction

Oxalates also have a significant effect on your brain. Oxalate trouble can manifest itself as neurological problems. The nerve irritation caused by them can manifest as hiccups. Reducing your intake of oxalates can eliminate sleep problems, emotional and mental fatigue, inability to concentrate, neuropathic pain, and cognitive issues. Accumulation of oxalates in the motor nerves results in muscle weakness, tremors, unsteadiness, twitching, and lack of coordination. Skin sensitivity and carpal tunnel syndrome can be a result of oxalate poisoning. By reducing your intake of oxalate-rich foods in your daily diet, the toxic damage to neurons can be reduced.

Deal with Urogenital Problems

Excess presence of oxalates in the body can result in urogenital problems such as bladder or urethral pain, frequent urination, urinary urgency, kidney pain, kidney stones, weakened pelvic floor, prostatitis, and even occasional incontinence. Accumulation of oxalates is believed to be the leading cause of kidney stones. Since kidneys are responsible for eliminating oxalates from blood, a high concentration of oxalates disrupts the kidneys' usual functioning. Any sensitivity, pain, inflammation, or tenderness in external and internal genitalia can also be a sign of oxalate accumulation. To restore the kidney's health and functioning, a low-oxalate diet comes in handy.

Better Nutrition

Oxalate acid not only combines with calcium, but it also absorbs iron, magnesium, and other metallic nutrients your body needs. When all these essential nutrients are combined with oxalates, your body does not absorb them, so even if your diet is rich in these micronutrients, their nutritional benefits are not available. In the long run, a deficiency of these nutrients occurs. Oxalate buildup can also trigger a vitamin B deficiency. Oxalates tend to absorb the vitamin B-6 present in the body. When the levels of this vitamin reduce, it increases the production of oxalates. This is a vicious cycle that leads to vitamin B deficiency while increasing the presence of oxalates. If left unchecked, it can result in oxalate poisoning and all the conditions mentioned above.

Sustainable in The Long Run

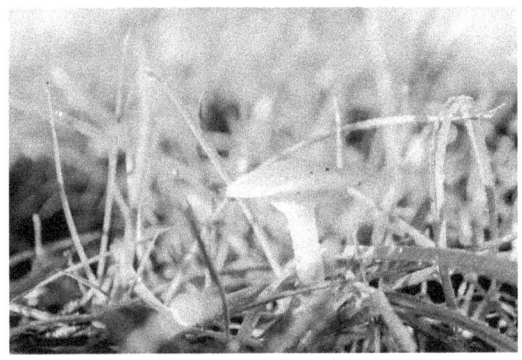

A significant benefit of the low-oxalate diet is it is sustainable in the long run. Unlike most other fad diets, which promise quick results, the oxalate diet isn't a short-term solution. Instead, it is a simple lifestyle change that is maintainable in the long run. As long as you follow this diet's simple protocols, you can continue to reap all the benefits it offers. Also, this diet isn't restrictive and is inclusive. All you need to do is carefully go through the different low-oxalate diet food list in the next section and stick to it.

By now, you will have realized the low-oxalate diet not only reduces the risk of kidney stones but helps improve your overall health. So, all that's left for you to do is get started with this diet!

OXALATE DIET FOOD LIST

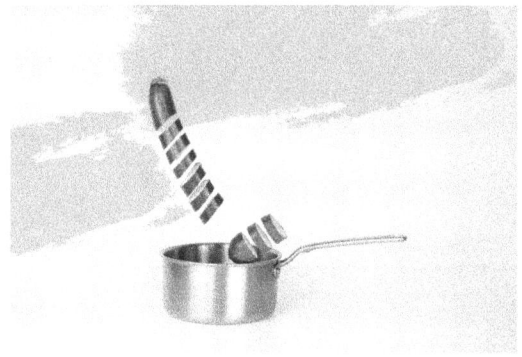

Are you wondering what you can and cannot eat on this diet? The diet is not restrictive and is inclusive. You merely need to avoid high-oxalate foods, limit your intake of moderate-oxalate foods, and feast on low-oxalate foods. This food list will come in handy while shopping for groceries. Don't forget to eliminate all high-oxalate foods from your pantry before starting this diet to eliminate any temptations.

HIGH-OXALATE FOODS TO AVOID

Vegetables

- Green Beans
- Beetroot
- Beet Greens
- Carrots
- Collard Greens
- Celery
- Chicory
- Dandelion Greens
- Chili Peppers
- Green Peppers
- Pokeweed
- Eggplant
- Okra
- Leeks
- Escarole
- Parsley
- Olives
- Potato

- Swiss Chard
- Summer Squash
- Spinach
- Zucchini
- Rutabaga
- Sweet Potato

Fruits

- Blackberries
- Currants
- Dewberries
- Blueberries
- Carambola
- Canned Strawberries
- Concord grape
- Tamarillo
- Tangerines
- Elderberries
- Figs
- Raspberries
- Orange, Lime, and Lemon Peels
- Fruit Cocktail
- Rhubarb
- Kiwis

Starches

- Buckwheat
- Amaranth
- Bran and Other High-Fiber Cereals
- Rye or Wheat Bread
- Taro

- Wheat Bran
- Wheat Germ
- Whole Wheat Bread and Flour
- Pretzels
- Grits

Dairy Products

- Chocolate Milk
- Soy Milk
- Soy Cheese
- Soy Yogurt

Fats, Nuts, and Seeds

- All Nuts and Nut Butter
- Sesame Seeds and Tahini
- Soy nuts

Beverages

- Instant Coffee
- Soy Drinks
- Cocoa and Chocolate Milk
- Juices Made with High-Oxalate Fruits
- Black Tea
- Dark Beer

Condiments

- Black Pepper
- Soy Sauce
- Marmalade

Miscellaneous Items

- Parsley and Chocolate

Note: The high-oxalate foods discussed in this section contain more than 10 mg of oxalate, so these are the items you must avoid.

LIMIT THE INTAKE OF MODERATE-OXALATE FOODS

Vegetables

- Asparagus
- Fennel
- Artichoke
- Brussels sprout
- Broccoli
- Lettuce
- Mustard Greens
- Carrots
- Corn
- Onions
- Parsnip
- Lima Beans
- Tomatoes
- Canned Peas
- Tomatoes and Vegetable Soup
- Watercress

Fruits

- Apples
- Apricots
- Applesauce
- Cranberries
- Coconut
- Oranges
- Mandarin
- Fresh Peaches
- Pineapple
- Fresh pear
- Prunes
- Fresh Strawberries
- Plums

Starches

- Bagels
- Corn Starch
- Cornmeal
- Brown Rice
- Oatmeal
- White Bread
- Corn Tortillas
- Pop-Tarts
- Sponge Cake

Meats

- Liver
- Sardines

Dairy Products

- Yogurt

Fats, Nuts, and Seeds

- Sunflower Seeds and Flaxseeds

Beverages

- Carrot Juice
- Brewed Coffee
- Grape Juice
- Cranberry Juice
- Orange Juice
- Tomato Juice
- Draft and Guinness Draft Beer

Miscellaneous Items

- Potato Chips
- Ginger
- Thyme
- Malt
- Strawberry Preserves and Jams

Note: Make sure that you don't consume more than 2-3 servings of these foods daily. Moderate-oxalate foods tend to have 2-10 mg of oxalate per serving.

INCREASE THE INTAKE OF LOW-OXALATE FOODS AND BEVERAGES

Vegetables

- Cucumber
- Cauliflower
- Cabbage
- Peas
- Kohlrabi
- Chives
- Endives
- Mushrooms
- Water Chestnuts
- Radishes

Fruits

- Avocados
- Bananas
- Cherries
- Grapefruit
- Huckleberries

- Red and Green Grapes
- Lychees
- Kumquat
- Nectarines
- Mangoes
- Papaya
- Melons
- Yellow and Green Plums
- Passion Fruit
- Canned Pears and Peaches

Starches

- Barley
- Corn and Rice Cereals
- Graham Crackers
- Egg Noodles
- English Muffin
- White Rice
- Wild Rice
- Pasta

Meats

- Bacon
- Ham
- Pork
- Poultry
- All Fish Except Sardines
- Shellfish
- Beef
- Corned Beef
- Lamb

- All Lean Meats

Dairy Products

- Milk
- Cheese
- Buttermilk

Fats, Nuts, and Seeds

- Butter
- Margarine
- Vegetable Oil
- Salad Dressing
- Mayonnaise

Beverages

- Herbal Teas
- Lime Juice
- Lemonade
- Oolong Tea
- Lemon Juice
- Green Tea
- Grapefruit Juice
- Apple Juice
- Buttermilk
- Apple Cider
- Apricot Nectar
- Bottled Beer
- Cherry Juice
- Pineapple Juice

Condiments

- Basil
- White Paper
- Vinegar
- Sugar
- Sage
- Peppermint
- Honey
- Cinnamon
- Dill
- Dijon Mustard
- Nutmeg
- Oregano
- Corn syrup
- Vanilla Extract
- Maple Syrup
- Ketchup (Not More than a Tbsp)
- Any Jelly Made with Low-Oxalate Fruits
- Any Other Dried Herbs

Miscellaneous Items

- Unflavored Gelatin
- Jell-O
- Hard Candy
- Lemon Balm

Note: The low-oxalate foods discussed in the section contain less than 2 mg of oxalate per serving so you can consume as much of these low oxalate foods as you want.

GETTING STARTED WITH THE LOW-OXALATE DIET

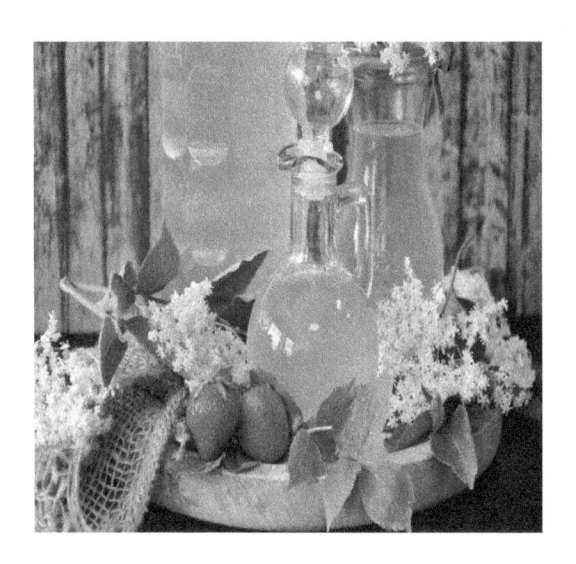

Getting started with the low-oxalate diet is a wonderful idea for your health. It is the simplest way to reverse several painful and harmful health conditions. Now that you are eager to get started with this diet, here are a few useful tips that will come in handy.

TIPS TO FOLLOW AND MISTAKES TO AVOID

Never dive headfirst into a diet without knowing what it's about. Lack of proper understanding and misinformation seldom offer good results. You can learn a lot from experience, but you can also learn from others' mistakes. In this section, let's look at the common mistakes you should avoid and the right practices to follow to increase the low oxalate diet's success.

Lack of Sufficient Hydration

Dehydration causes a variety of issues ranging from poor skin health to improper digestion. It can also trigger headaches and increase the risk of kidney stones. The recommended intake of water for an adult is 2-3 liters per day. You need to consume enough water to keep your body functioning optimally. The simplest way to make sure you consume sufficient water is by carrying a water bottle with you. Take it with you everywhere you go and sip from it regularly. You can add a couple of slices of lime or mint leaves to spruce up regular water. Hydrate your body regularly to improve your overall health. Also, this is the key to healthy, supple, and youthful skin.

Avoid Eating Out

Since we all lead busy lives, it can be quite tempting to eat out or order takeout. Resist the urge to do this. It might help save time and effort, but in the long run, it harms your health. Even meals that are labeled as healthy are not truly healthy. Instead of burning a hole in your pocket by eating out, it is always better to cook meals at home. Most restaurants use a lot of salt in their food. High levels of sodium can hamper kidney functioning and increase the risk of stone formation. Even if you get a healthy meal at a restaurant, chances are it is loaded with salt. Avoid eating foods rich in sodium and monitor your salt intake. The ideal intake of sodium must not exceed 2300 mg for an entire day. This limit is even lower if you are at the risk of developing kidney stones.

You don't have to spend hours together in the kitchen to cook a healthy and nutritious meal. All the different recipes given in this book are incredibly simple to follow and wholesome. You merely need to stock your pantry with low oxalate foods and select a recipe that strikes your fancy. Yes, this is about it. It's not just your body that will be grateful for home-cooked meals, but your bank balance will be happy too.

Improper Hydration

Drinking water is important, but it is also important to hydrate your body properly. Improper hydration does you no good. For instance, consuming energy drinks or sports drinks might help meet your daily water requirement, but they are also filled with sodium that your body doesn't need. You can also obtain water from fresh fruit juices. That said, drinking juices made of high-oxalate fruits is counterintuitive. When in doubt, opt for regular water! Also, try to eliminate pre-packaged and processed juices and beverages if you want to improve your overall health. The hidden sugars, preservatives, and added sodium do more harm than good.

Don't Drink Alkaline Water

Several people believe drinking alkaline water can increase your metabolism, slow down the aging process, and even prevent diseases, but it is important to note that these claims don't have any scientific backing or validation so avoid drinking alkaline water. Even if you want to do this, it is always advisable that you consult your healthcare provider. There have been instances where excessive consumption of alkaline water is associated with serious kidney stones.

Pay Attention to Your Calcium Intake

It is important to monitor your calcium intake. Remember, oxalates tend to bind with calcium in the body. Unbound oxalates are quite dangerous. If you reduce your calcium intake, it increases the risk of the presence of unbound oxalates. Also, calcium is important for maintaining bone health. By reducing your calcium intake, you are essentially increasing the risk of kidney stones. When oxalate binds with calcium, it is eliminated from your body. When there is no calcium, oxalate buildup increases and results in kidney stones, so always opt for a well-rounded diet that caters to your body's calcium requirements.

Avoid High Oxalate Foods

A common mistake many people make while trying to reduce their risk of kidney stones is that they concentrate only on their calcium intake. Regulating your calcium intake is important, but your primary focus should be to reduce your oxalate intake. Since oxalate is produced by your body and is found in several types of plant-based foods, it is easy to go overboard. If left unregulated, high levels of oxalate in the body can result in different problems discussed in the previous chapter. Instead of doing all this, it's better to follow a low-oxalate diet. Concentrate on avoiding high oxalate foods and increase your intake of low-oxalate foods. A detailed list of the different foods you can and cannot eat has been discussed in the previous chapter, so ensure you carefully go through it and stock your pantry with the required ingredients.

Using Supplements with Unknown Ingredients

A popular misconception is that all supplements are created equally. Supplements don't necessarily mean a healthier you. The human body requires a variety of nutrients and micronutrients for it to function optimally. Taking a supplement can ensure that your body gets its daily dose of nutrients. It only needs a certain amount of nutrients, and beyond that, the nutrients don't serve a purpose. Before you take a supplement, make sure you carefully go through the list of ingredients. For instance, a supplement with spinach extract is not advisable for anyone who wants to follow a low oxalate diet. Spinach is rich in oxalates, and it increases the chances of all the health problems associated with oxalate concentration. Before you start taking the supplement, don't forget to consult your healthcare provider.

Monitor Your Protein Intake

By following a low-oxalate diet, you can eat various types of animal proteins except for liver and sardines, but excess consumption of animal protein can increase the risk of kidney stones. Ideally, around 10-35% of your daily calories should be from proteins such as meat, seafood, legumes, and poultry. Try to stay within this limit if you want to improve your overall health. For more information, go through the food list discussed in the previous chapter.

Giving Up Too Soon

A common mistake many people make while shifting to a new diet is that they expect immediate results. If you want this diet to be successful, you need to follow it for 3-4 weeks, at least. It is not a magic pill that can solve your problems. Instead, it is a long-term solution that improves your overall health and reduces the occurrence of the harmful conditions associated with oxalate buildup. Ensure that you strictly follow the protocols of this diet and don't stray away from it. Learn to be patient with yourself. Starting a new diet is a significant change for your body, and it will take time to get used to it. Don't be under any misimpression that it will be easy. Since you will be eliminating common foods, getting accustomed to it takes time. Be patient and compassionate towards your body if you want to see a positive change.

Don't Forget to Consume a Diverse Diet

Don't be under any misconceptions that the low-oxalate diet is restrictive. Instead, it merely suggests you need to avoid all high-oxalate ingredients. If your diet is too repetitive or boring, the chances that you will give up on it increase. A simple way to ensure that you stick to this diet, in the long run, is by making it diverse. Don't consume similar meals daily and add variety. The good news is you don't have to spend hours together searching for low-oxalate diet recipes. All the recipes you need are provided in this book. Go through the different recipes, create a meal plan that works for you, and stick to it.

Set Realistic Goals

Before you start this diet, it is important to set certain goals. Goals tend to provide a sense of purpose and direction in life. They ensure you are heading in the right direction and are making progress. Without goals, the chances of failure increase. Well, the same applies to any diet you follow. So, it is time to set goals. While setting goals, make sure they are small, measure able, attainable, relevant, and time-bound. Even if one of these ingredients is missing, the chances of attaining the goal will reduce. A simple goal you can set for yourself is to follow the low-oxalate diet for a week. Once you follow it for a week, set a goal that you will follow for two weeks, and so on. Whenever you attain a goal, it increases your self-confidence and gives you the internal motivation required to keep going. The progress you make is also a motivating factor. If you follow this diet for at least a month, you will see a positive change in your overall health.

Avoid Temptations

While following a diet, you need to remember a simple tip is "out of sight, out of mind." Before you start the low-oxalate diet, spend time, and go through your pantry. Get rid of all temptations, especially foods rich in oxalates. If you are constantly surrounded by temptations, the chances of straying from the diet increase. By stocking your pantry with low-oxalate diet ingredients, cooking also becomes easier. Think of it as spring-cleaning, where you are eliminating all traces of unhealthy foods from your home.

An Occasional Slipup isn't A Failure

Do not hold on to a perfectionist attitude when it comes to a diet. Prepare yourself for an occasional slipup. By viewing an occasional slipup as a failure, the chances that you will give up on the diet increase. For instance, if you binge on any high-oxalate foods, get back to your diet from the following day. An all-or-nothing attitude prevents you from doing this. It also increases the chances of abandoning the diet altogether.

Create a Plan

Before you start the diet, you need a plan of action. Spend time, go through the different recipes given in this book, shop for the required groceries, and create a meal plan. Over the weekend, spend time on meal prepping. If all the ingredients are prepped and ready, cooking a meal becomes incredibly simple. All it takes is a few hours on the weekend to do the essential meal prep for the meals you wish to cook in the upcoming week. When you know fresh, healthy, delicious, and nutritious meals are waiting for you at home, the temptation to eat out decreases. A little planning and preparation increase your chances of success.

Have A Support System

Following a new diet isn't always easy. Even if your motivation levels are quite high initially, as the weeks go by, the likelihood that they will decrease is high. Remember, you might not be able to see any positive results immediately. It doesn't mean the diet isn't working. It takes a while for the positive change to become visible. Meanwhile, you need to ensure that you follow this diet strictly. Before starting the diet, make sure you have a support system in place. Your support system can consist of family members, loved ones, or colleagues.

Why do you need a support system? A support system ensures that you follow this diet. The odds that you will stick to the diet increase when you know you are accountable to someone else. This added responsibility increases your chances of success. If you want, you can reach out to others online. These days, there are several online platforms and chat rooms you can participate in to interact with others who follow a low-oxalate diet. When you know others are going through the same situation you are experiencing right now, it will make you feel better. When you interact with others, chances are, you will stumble upon helpful tips and other insights.

By following the simple tips and advice given in this section, getting accustomed to the low oxalate diet becomes easy.

Note: If you have any pre-existing medical conditions or health problems, always consult your doctor before making any dietary changes. If you have recently undergone major surgery or will undergo one in the future, it is especially important to get your doctor's consent. This is the same rule you need to follow before you start taking any supplements too.

MYTHS ABOUT LOW-OXALATE DIET

Oxalates are highly reactive molecules, and they tend to bind themselves with minerals such as calcium, magnesium, iron, and copper. It is important to equip yourself with the right information before you start a diet. Whenever a diet gains popularity, several misconceptions about it start cropping up. Following the wrong diet or improper dietary protocols do your body more harm than good. In this section, let's look at common myths associated with a low oxalate diet.

Myth #1: Cooked High-Oxalate Food Is Safe

A common myth about high oxalate foods is that the oxalate in them is destroyed when cooked. To a certain extent, this is true. Cooking methods such as boiling the ingredients and then immediately dumping them in cold water reduces the oxalate present in them, but sautéing, baking, and steaming are other cooking methods that are not that effective. Even if broiling or boiling reduces the ingredients' oxalates, the reduction is only about 50% so if a high oxalate food such as spinach contains 500 mg of oxalate, boiling it will reduce it only to 250 mg. This is still too high for your body. Instead of making high oxalate foods safer for consumption, it's better to increase your low-oxalate foods intake.

Myth #2: All Oxalates Are Bad

Balance is needed in all aspects of your life, and health is not an exception. Math states that every function has a limit. Similarly, recognize the limits of your physical body while concentrating on improving your health. In regulated amounts, oxalates are good. Only when their concentration increases do they become harmful. So, don't be under the misconception that all oxalates are bad and need to be eliminated. If you concentrate on quickly eliminating all oxalates or remove them quickly, it can cause physical symptoms due to oxalate dumping. Instead, you need to slowly stabilize the oxalate levels to the extent that it is tolerable for your body.

Myth #3: Spinach Is A Superfood And Must Be Good For You

Food is the source of nutrition and helps sustain your body. It can heal, but consuming the wrong foods can wreak havoc on your health. Certain foods such as spinach are considered superfoods because they are a powerhouse of nutrients and minerals your body needs. Unfortunately, spinach is also rich in oxalates. Do you see how something that can be good can also be bad?

Spinach is rich in calcium and folate. Both of these ingredients are helpful for your body, but the calcium present in it is bound to the oxalates it contains, so if you eat spinach, all the helpful calcium is not available for your body to be absorbed. In a way, you are merely increasing your intake of oxalates and nothing more. Instead of worrying about eliminating spinach, opt for low-oxalate foods that are rich in calcium and folate. Just because it's a superfood doesn't mean it's good for you.

Myth 4#: A Health Microbiome Means You Don't Have To Worry About Oxalates

The gut microbiome ensures that your gut functions optimally, so it is important to fix your gut microbiome. When it comes to balancing your gut microbiome and stabilizing oxalates, there is a vicious cycle that not many are aware of. Oxalates damage the functioning of healthy bacteria and even destroy the equilibrium of the gut microbiome. If the gut microbiome is not functioning as required, it increases the levels of oxalates. This is the vicious cycle you need to avoid. If you want to improve your overall health, you need healthy gut flora and low oxalate levels. So, don't be under the wrong impression that improving your gut microbiome will automatically fix the oxalate levels. It is important to follow the low-oxalate diet, and you cannot do away with it if you want your health to improve. Also, it is incredibly difficult to fix the gut microbiome if your oxalate levels are quite high. You need a two-pronged approach to fix this situation.

Myth 5#: Eliminating Yeast Helps Reduce Oxalate Levels

A common myth is that oxalates are caused by yeast or Candida, so this suggests that eliminating yeast can reduce oxalate levels. There might be a correlation between yeast overgrowth, oxalates, and oxalate dumping, but there is no scientific evidence that suggests that Candida produces oxalates in the body. Controlling yeast levels and balancing the gut microbial are important and can reduce oxalate issues, but these are not the only factors that need to be considered. It is important to follow a low-oxalate diet if you want to regulate your oxalate levels and bring them under control.

Myth #6: Inability To Handle Oxalates Suggests Oxalate Intolerance

If your body cannot handle oxalates, it doesn't mean you have an oxalate intolerance or oxalate and sensitivity. The problem with oxalates is it is not a food allergy or sensitivity. It is also not an immune system problem, so labeling it as intolerance is highly incorrect. Intolerance essentially implies that an individual isn't able to tolerate oxalate for a specific reason, but the human body is adept at tolerating oxalates in regulated amounts. The problem starts only when the oxalate levels are too high for you to manage.

During the initial few days of the diet, you might feel worse than before. This is usually a sign of oxalate dumping. Remember, Rome wasn't built in a day. When it comes to a diet, you need to opt for a sustainable eating protocol. Instead of eliminating all oxalate forms from your diet in one go, opt for a slow process.

Myth #7: Greens Are Healthy. A Low-Oxalate Diet Is Devoid Of All Healthy Greens

Another myth you need to be wary of is that all greens are rich in oxalates. Don't worry that there will be no healthy greens left in your diet if you follow a low oxalate diet. Several healthy greens are low in oxalates such as bok choy, arugula, alfalfa sprouts, cabbage, turnip and dandelion greens, dinosaur kale, and romaine lettuce. You can easily obtain all the nutrients your body needs, even while following a low-oxalate diet. The only thing you need to remember is to consume healthy and wholesome meals based on the low-oxalate diet food list.

Myth #8: Grains Are Bad For Gut And Inflammatory Bowel Conditions Benefit From Nut Flours

If you have a sensitive digestive system or any pre-existing gut issues, consuming grains can be problematic. This essentially means that all such individuals usually turn to nut flours. Nut flours might not necessarily be the best option. Since they contain high levels of oxalate, they can worsen any gut issues or cause new issues. If your digestive system is sensitive, you should consult your healthcare provider before adding or eliminating certain foods from your diet.

Myth #9: A Low-Oxalate Diet Means You Have No Issues With Oxalate

Oxalates are created endogenously and are present in different types of foods too. Consuming a low oxalate diet doesn't necessarily mean you have no oxalate issues. Instead, it merely helps stabilize the levels of oxalate in your body. High oxalate levels are problematic, and once these levels are within control, your body can deal with it. Since your body produces oxalates internally, the diet you consume needs to account for this proportion too.

Myth #10: More Calcium Means You Don't Have To Follow A Low-Oxalate Diet

A common misconception about the low oxalate diet is that consumption of excess calcium is good. It is based on the wrong notion that more calcium means you don't have to follow a low oxalate diet. Oxalates bind with calcium, but it is important to remember that your body also produces oxalates. It essentially means that your body already has more oxalates than calcium present in it can handle. You must remember that foods rich in oxalates don't necessarily have enough calcium, which ensures that all the oxalate molecules are bound together. The simple takeaway is to remember you cannot counter the presence of oxalates with calcium alone.

RECIPES

EGGLESS PANCAKES

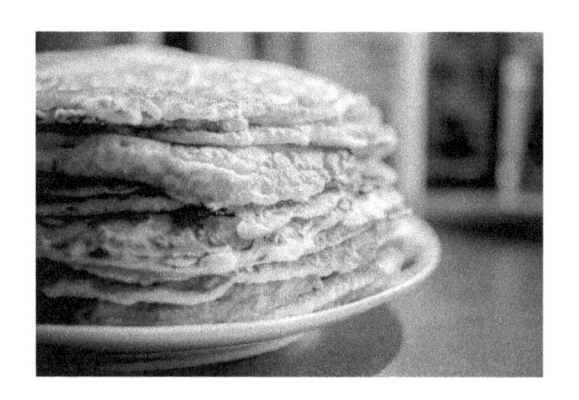

Serves: 3

Nutritional values per serving: 1 pancake, without toppings

Calories – 157

Fat – 7.2 g

Total Carbohydrate – 19.5 g

Protein – 3.5 g

Ingredients:

- ½ cup all-purpose flour
- 1/8 teaspoon ground cinnamon
- 1/8 teaspoon salt
- ½ tablespoon vegetable oil
- ½ teaspoon vanilla extract
- ½ teaspoon sugar
- 1 teaspoon baking powder
- ½ cup milk
- ½ tablespoon water
- 1 tablespoon butter

Directions:

1. Combine flour, cinnamon, salt, baking powder, and sugar in a bowl.
2. Combine milk, vegetable oil, vanilla, and water in another bowl. Pour the milk mixture into the bowl of flour mixture and stir until well combined, making sure not to over-mix. Let it rest for 5 minutes.
3. Place a griddle pan over medium flame and let it heat.
4. Add 1/3-tablespoon butter and let it melt. Pour 1/3 of the batter. In a couple of minutes, bubbles will be visible on top of the pancake.
5. Cook until the underside is golden brown. Turn the pancake over and cook the other side as well. Remove pancake from the pan and serve with toppings of your choice.
6. Repeat steps 4 – 5 and make the remaining pancakes.

CHIVE & GOAT CHEESE SOUFFLÉS

Serves: 8

Nutritional values per serving:

Calories – 252

Fat – 18 g

Carbohydrates – 9 g

Protein – 14 g

Ingredients:

- 1 cup grated, packed Parmesan cheese, divided
- 4 tablespoons butter
- 2 cups low- fat milk
- ¼ teaspoon salt
- 8 large eggs, separated
- 2/3 cup minced, fresh chives, divided
- 5 tablespoons all-purpose flour
- ½ teaspoon pepper

- 4 ounces soft goat's cheese, at room temperature, crumbled
- 1 teaspoon grated lemon zest

Directions:

1. Prepare 8 ramekins (10 ounces each) by greasing them with cooking spray.
2. Scatter a teaspoon of Parmesan and ½ teaspoon chives on the bottom of each of the ramekins.
3. Place a saucepan over medium flame. Add butter. Once butter melts, add flour and constantly stir for about 30 seconds.
4. Add milk, salt, and pepper. Stir constantly until thick. Turn off the heat.
5. Add goat's cheese, remaining chives, and Parmesan cheese. Whisk well.
6. Add an egg yolk at a time and whisk each time. Add zest and stir.
7. Add whites into another bowl. Whisk using an electric hand mixer until stiff peaks are just beginning to form.
8. Pour 1/3 of the whites into the souffle batter. Fold gently. Pour batter into the prepared ramekins (add equal quantities in each).
9. Place the ramekins on a rimmed baking sheet.
10. Place the ramekins along with the baking sheet in an oven that has been preheated to 375°F and bake until brown on top. It should take around 20 – 25 minutes.

BELGIAN WAFFLES

Serves: 4

Nutritional values per serving: 1 waffle, without toppings

Calories – 391

Fat – 17 g

Total Carbohydrate – 35 g

Protein – 6 g

Ingredients:

- 1 1/8 cups all-purpose flour
- 1 ½ tablespoons sugar
- ½ teaspoon ground cinnamon
- ¼ cup vegetable oil
- ½ teaspoon vanilla extract
- ½ tablespoon baking powder
- ¼ teaspoon salt
- 1 large egg, separated
- 1 cup milk

Directions:

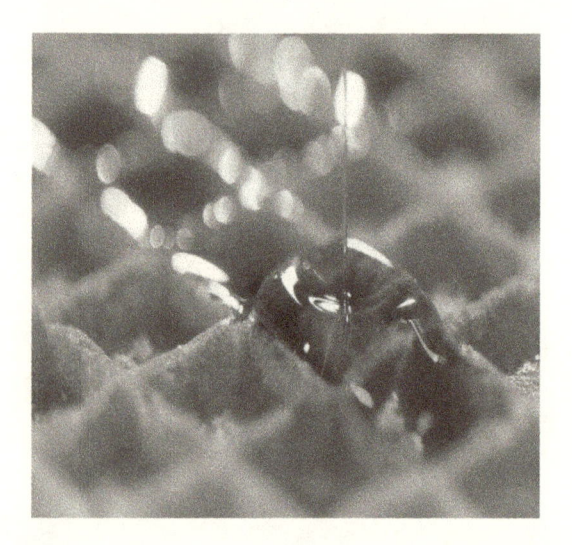

1. Combine flour, cinnamon, salt, baking powder, and sugar in a bowl.
2. Using an electric hand mixer, beat the egg white until stiff peaks are formed.
3. Combine yolk, vegetable oil, vanilla, and milk in another bowl. Pour the milk mixture into the bowl of flour mixture and stir until well combined, making sure not to over-mix.
4. Add egg white and fold gently.
5. Plug in your waffle iron and allow it to preheat, following the directions of the manufacturer.
6. Spray cooking spray on the iron.
7. Pour ¼ of the batter into the waffle iron. Close the lid and set the timer for 4 – 6 minutes, depending on how you like it cooked. Remove the waffle and place on a plate.

8. Repeat the previous step and make the other waffle.
9. Serve with toppings of your choice.

EASY TUNA PASTA SALAD

Serves: 4

Nutritional values per serving:

Calories – 557.1

Fat – 27.2 g

Total Carbohydrate – 53.6 g

Protein – 26.4 g

Ingredients:

- 8 ounces Cavatappi (corkscrew macaroni)
- 1 ½ tablespoons lemon juice
- ¾ teaspoon garlic powder
- 1 can (8 ounces) tuna, drained
- ½ red onion, diced
- 2 tablespoons chopped parsley
- ½ teaspoon lemon juice or to taste
- ½ cup mayonnaise
- 1 tablespoon honey

- Salt to taste
- Pepper to taste
- 1 ½ stalks celery, diced
- ½ cup peas
- ¼ cup chopped green olives
- 2 hard-boiled eggs, peeled, quartered

Directions:

1. Cook pasta until a minute before the time mentioned on the instructions on the package.

2. Place drained pasta into a bowl.

3. Add tuna, onion, parsley, celery, peas, and olives and toss well.

4. To make the dressing: Add mayonnaise, honey, salt, lemon juice, garlic powder, and pepper into a small bowl and whisk well. Cover and set aside for a while for the flavors to blend in.

5. Add dressing into the bowl of salad and fold gently.

6. Divide the salad onto 4 plates. Place ½ boiled egg (2 quarters) on each and serve.

CORDON BLEU SALAD

Serves: 4

Nutritional values per serving:

Calories – 965.4

Fat – 66.3 g

Total Carbohydrate – 60.8 g

Protein – 33.9 g

Ingredients:

For Salad:

- 8 ounces farfalle pasta (bowtie pasta)
- 1 cup cubed, cooked ham
- ½ cup broccoli florets
- 1 cup cooked, cubed chicken
- 1 cup cubed Swiss cheese

For Dressing:

- 2 tablespoons honey
- 1 tablespoon Dijon mustard
- 1 tablespoon chopped onion
- 2 tablespoons white sugar
- 1 tablespoon chopped parsley
- ¾ cup mayonnaise
- 1 tablespoons white vinegar
- ¼ cup olive oil
- ¼ teaspoon garlic salt
- 2 tablespoons grated Parmesan cheese

Directions:

1. Cook pasta until al dente, following the instructions on the package. Drain and set aside in a bowl.
2. Add ham, chicken, broccoli, and Swiss cheese and toss well.
3. To make the dressing: Add honey, mustard, onion, sugar, mayonnaise, vinegar, oil, and garlic salt into a blender and blend until smooth.
4. Add parsley and stir. Pour half the dressing into the salad and fold gently.
5. Refrigerate for a couple of hours.
6. Add remaining dressing and Parmesan cheese and fold gently.
7. Serve.

CHERRY TOMATO CORN SALAD

Serves: 3

Nutritional values per serving:

Calories – 138

Fat – 7.4 g

Total Carbohydrate – 18.4 g

Protein – 2.7 g

Ingredients:

For Dressing:

- 2 tablespoons minced fresh basil
- 1 teaspoon lime juice
- ¼ teaspoon salt
- 1 ½ tablespoons olive oil
- ½ teaspoon white sugar
- 1/8 teaspoon pepper

For Salad:

- 1 cup frozen corn, thawed
- ½ cup peeled, deseeded, chopped cucumber
- 1 shallot, minced
- 1 cup halved cherry tomatoes
- ½ jalapeno pepper, chopped

Directions:

1. To make the dressing: Add all the ingredients for dressing into a small jar. Fasten the lid and shake the jar vigorously until well combined.
2. To make the salad: Add all the ingredients for salad into a bowl and toss well.
3. Pour dressing over the salad. Toss well and chill until you serve.

TROPICAL TURKEY SALAD

Serves: 6

Nutritional values per serving:

Calories – 125.7

Fat – 3.2 g

Total Carbohydrate – 9.6 g

Protein – 14.4 g

Ingredients:

For Dressing:

- 1 tablespoon mango chutney
- ½ tablespoon honey
- ½ tablespoon fresh lemon juice
- 1/8 teaspoon curry powder

For Salad:

- ½ cup chopped onion
- 2 cups cooked, chopped turkey
- ½ cup diced celery
- ½ cup chopped orange segments
- ½ cup diced red bell pepper
- ½ cup pineapple chunks

Directions:

1. To make the dressing: Add mango chutney, honey, lemon juice, and curry powder into a small jar. Fasten the lid and shake the jar vigorously until well combined.
2. To make the salad: Add all the ingredients for salad into a bowl and toss well.
3. Pour dressing over the salad. Toss well and chill until you serve.

BEEF NOODLE SOUP

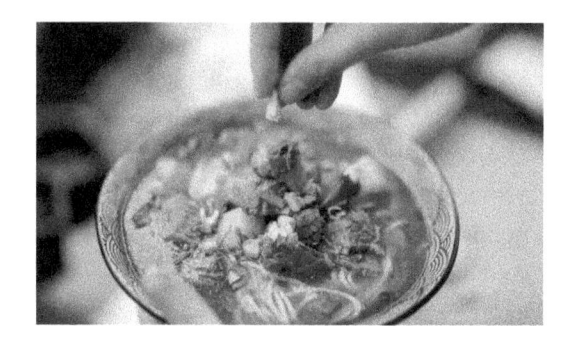

Serves: 3

Nutritional values per serving:

Calories – 377.2

Fat – 19.4 g

Total Carbohydrate – 24.8 g

Protein – 25.5 g

Ingredients:

- ½ pound cubed beef stew meat
- ½ cup chopped celery
- A large pinch dried celery
- ½ cup chopped carrots
- 1 ¼ cups frozen egg noodles
- ½ cup chopped onion
- 2 tablespoons beef bouillon granules
- Pepper to taste
- 2 ½ cups water or more if required

Directions:

1. Place a soup pot over medium-high flame. Add onion, beef, and celery and sauté until beef is brown all over.
2. Add parsley, bouillon, carrots, egg noodles, parsley, and pepper. When it begins to boil, lower the heat and cook on low for about 15 – 20 minutes or until meat and noodles are cooked.

ROASTED RED PEPPER AND POTATO SOUP

Serves: 3

Nutritional values per serving:

Calories – 204

Fat – 9 g

Total Carbohydrate – 26 g

Protein – 6 g

Ingredients:

- 1 medium onion, chopped
- ½ jar (from a 7 ounces jar) roasted sweet red peppers with its liquid, chopped
- 1 ½ cups peeled, chopped potatoes
- ½ teaspoon ground coriander
- ½ teaspoon salt to taste
- 1 teaspoon ground cumin
- 2 ounces canned, chopped green chilies, drained
- 1 ½ cups vegetable broth

- ½ tablespoon lemon juice
- A handful fresh cilantro, minced
- ¼ cup cubed low-fat cream cheese
- 1 tablespoon canola oil

Directions:

1. Place a soup pot over medium heat. Add oil. When the oil is heated, add onions and cook until translucent.
2. Add roasted red peppers, chilies, salt, cumin, and coriander and stir-fry for a couple of minutes.
3. Add potatoes and broth and cook until potatoes are soft. Turn off the heat.
4. Add lemon juice and cilantro and stir. Cool the soup for a while.
5. Transfer half the soup into a blender. Add cream cheese and blend until smooth.
6. Pour the blended soup back into the saucepan along with the remaining soup. Heat thoroughly.
7. Ladle into soup bowls and serve.

CHICKEN AND RICE SOUP

Serves: 8

Nutritional values per serving:

Calories – 504

Fat – 19 g

Total Carbohydrate – 57 g

Protein – 27 g

Ingredients:

- 1 pound onions, chopped
- ½ pound celery stalks, chopped
- 1 ½ pounds carrots, chopped
- 1 ½ pounds skinless, boneless chicken thighs
- 2 cups uncooked, medium-grain rice
- 2 teaspoons minced parsley
- 1 teaspoon dried thyme, divided
- 1 teaspoon salt, divided
- 8 tablespoons heavy cream

- 2 tablespoons olive oil
- 2 teaspoons minced garlic
- 2 teaspoons black pepper, divided
- 20 cups unsalted chicken broth
- 4 tablespoons unsalted butter

Directions:

1. Place a large soup pot over a medium flame. Add oil and let it heat.
2. Once the oil is heated, place chicken in the pot. Cook for 5 – 6 minutes. Sprinkle ½ teaspoon salt, ½ teaspoon thyme, and 1 teaspoon black pepper over the chicken and mix well.
3. Remove chicken with a slotted spoon and set aside on a plate lined with paper towels.
4. Add butter into the pot and allow it to melt.
5. Add onion and carrot and cook until onions turn pink.
6. Stir in celery, rice, and garlic. Stir frequently for a couple of minutes.
7. Pour broth and stir. Once the mixture comes to a boil, lower the heat and cook for about 30 – 35 minutes.
8. Blend lightly with an immersion blender. The soup should not be very smooth.
9. Stir in chicken, ½ teaspoon thyme, and ½ teaspoon salt and simmer for 2 – 3 minutes.
10. Finally goes in the cream. Stir until well combined.
11. Ladle into soup bowls. Garnish with parsley and remaining pepper and serve.

ZUCCHINI AND HALLOUMI BAKE

Serves: 3

Nutritional values per serving:

Calories – 1725

Fat – 47 g

Total Carbohydrate – 65 g

Protein – 141 g

Ingredients:

- 1 medium red onion
- A handful of fresh mint leaves
- A handful of fresh dill sprigs
- 1 tablespoon extra-virgin olive oil
- ½ tablespoon lemon juice
- 4 ounces halloumi, coarsely grated
- 6 tablespoons TLO low oxalate flour blend
- ½ tablespoon pine nuts

- 1 clove garlic, crushed
- 8.8 ounces zucchini, coarsely grated, squeezed of excess moisture
- 3 eggs
- ½ teaspoon baking powder
- Salt to taste
- 1/8 teaspoon sumac
- Pepper to taste

Directions:

1. Prepare a small, square baking dish by lining it with parchment paper, on the bottom as well as sides.
2. Cut 1/3 of the onion into thin round slices. Chop 2/3 of the onion into fine dice.
3. Retain a little of dill sprigs and mint leaves and finely chop the rest of it.
4. Place a pan over a medium-low flame. Add ½ tablespoon oil. When the oil is heated, add garlic and the finely diced onion. Once it turns pink, remove the onion-garlic mixture into a bowl.
5. Also add halloumi, zucchini, lemon juice, chopped dill, and mint and mix well.
6. Add eggs and ½ tablespoon oil into another bowl and whisk well.
7. Combine flour, salt, pepper, and baking powder and add into the bowl of eggs. Mix well.
8. Add into the bowl of zucchini mixture and stir well. Pour into the baking dish.
9. Scatter onion rings and retained dill sprigs and mint leaves.
10. Scatter pine and sumac on top.

11. Place the baking dish in an oven that has been preheated to 340°F and bake until cooked. It should take around 30 – 35 minutes. Let the bake remain in the baking dish for 10 minutes.
12. Slice and serve.

SPICY RANCH CAULIFLOWER CRACKERS

Serves: 36

Nutritional values per serving:

Calories – 28.6

Fat – 1.5 g

Total Carbohydrate – 1.3 g

Protein – 2.5 g

Ingredients:

- 2 packages (12 ounces each) frozen cauliflower rice
- 2 tablespoons dry ranch salad dressing mix
- 2 eggs
- ¼ teaspoon cayenne pepper or to taste

Directions:

1. Add cauliflower rice into a microwave-safe

container. Cook covered, in a microwave for 4 minutes.
2. Line a strainer with cheesecloth and add the cauliflower rice into it. Let it cool for about 20 minutes.
3. Bring together the edges of the cheesecloth together and squeeze out the moisture from the cauliflower.
4. Prepare a large baking sheet by lining with parchment paper. Use 2 baking sheets if required.
5. Add eggs, cayenne pepper, and ranch dressing mix into the bowl of cauliflower and mix until well combined.
6. Add Parmesan and mix well.
7. Make 36 equal portions of the mixture and place them on the baking sheet. Leave a sufficient gap between them.
8. Using the back of a glass or cup, flatten the cauliflower mixture until it is about 1/16 inch thick.
9. Place the baking sheet in an oven that has been preheated to 375°F and bake until brown. Flip sides after about 10 minutes and bake until crisp. It should take 20 – 30 minutes.

BROCCOLI WITH GARLIC AND CHILI

Serves: 3

Nutritional values per serving: 1/3 recipe

Calories – 142.9

Fat – 10 g

Total Carbohydrate – 1 g

Protein – 9 g

Ingredients:

- 14.1 ounces broccoli, cut into florets
- 2 cloves garlic, thinly sliced
- 1 tablespoon olive oil
- ¼ teaspoon salt
- ¼ teaspoon dried chili flakes
- Pepper to taste

Directions:

1. Place a pot of water over a high flame. When water begins to boil, add broccoli and cook until it turns bright green.
2. Drain the broccoli in a colander.
3. Place a pan over a medium flame. Add oil. Once the oil is heated, add garlic and cook for about 30 seconds, stirring constantly.
4. Stir in chili. Add broccoli after 5 – 8 seconds. Mix well. Add salt and pepper and toss well.
5. Divide onto 3 plates and serve.

BAKED BANANA CHIPS

Serves: 4

Nutritional values per serving:

Calories – 105.7

Fat – 0.4 g

Total Carbohydrate – 27.2 g

Protein – 1.3 g

Ingredients:

- 2 teaspoons lemon juice
- 4 just-ripe bananas, peeled, cut into 1/10 inch thick round slices

Directions:

1. Prepare a large baking sheet by lining with parchment paper.

2. Place the banana slices in a single layer without overlapping or even touching each other.
3. Brush lemon juice over the banana slices.
4. Place the baking sheet in an oven that has been preheated to 255°F and bake until crisp. Flip sides after every 60 minutes. It should take about 2 hours.
5. Remove the baking sheet from the oven and let it cool.
6. Transfer into an airtight container. It can last for 4 – 5 days.

GREEN BEANS, GROUND TURKEY AND RICE

Serves: 2

Nutritional values per serving:

Calories – 326

Fat – 15 g

Total Carbohydrate – 25 g

Protein – 25 g

Ingredients:

- ½ tablespoon + ½ teaspoon sesame oil
- 2 ½ cups green beans, trimmed
- ¾ cup cooked brown rice
- Freshly ground pepper to taste
- ½ pound 93% lean ground turkey
- Salt to taste

Directions:

1. Place a skillet over medium-high flame. Add oil. When the oil is heated, add turkey and cook until brown. Stir in green beans. Cover and cook until green beans are crisp as well as tender.
2. Sprinkle salt and pepper to taste.
3. Divide rice onto plates. Divide turkey and green beans among the plates and serve.

GRILLED PORK CHOPS WITH TWO-MELON SALSA

Serves: 8

Nutritional values per serving:

Calories – 256

Fat – 13.5 g

Total Carbohydrate – 8.7 g

Protein – 25 g

Ingredients:

For Salsa:

- 2 cups seedless watermelon
- 2 tablespoons jalapeno pepper, finely chopped
- 2 cups honeydew melon
- 1 large sweet onion, finely chopped
- 2 tablespoons chopped fresh cilantro
- 2 tablespoons fresh lime juice
- Salt to taste

For Pork Chops:

- 8 pork chops (4 ounces each) center-cut pork chops, boneless, trimmed of fat
- 4 teaspoons canola oil
- 1 teaspoon garlic powder
- 2 teaspoons chili powder
- Freshly ground pepper to taste
- Salt to taste

Directions:

1. To make the salsa: Mix watermelon, honeydew melon, jalapeño, onion, cilantro, lime juice, and salt in a bowl. Cover and set aside.
2. To make the pork chops: Set up your grill and preheat it to medium-high heat.
3. Mix in a bowl oil, garlic powder, chili powder, pepper, and salt. Rub this mixture over the pork chops.
4. Grill the pork for 4 minutes per side or until cooked as per your liking. Spray the chops with cooking spray while cooking.
5. Serve pork chops with the melon salsa.

PORK MEDALLIONS WITH GRAINY MUSTARD SAUCE

Serves: 2

Nutritional values per serving: 3 ounces pork with 2 tablespoons sauce

Calories – 200

Fat – 9.5 g

Total Carbohydrate – 2 g

Protein – 26 g

Ingredients:

- ½ tablespoon olive oil
- ¼ teaspoon salt, divided
- ¾ tablespoon Dijon mustard
- ¼ cup unsalted chicken stock
- ½ pound pork tenderloin, cut into 4 slices crosswise
- ¼ teaspoon freshly ground pepper
- ½ tablespoon unsalted butter
- ½ teaspoon all-purpose flour

Directions:

1. Place a skillet with oil over medium-high flame. Swirl the pan so that oil spreads.
2. Place pork slices in between your palms, one at a time, and press gently until flat.
3. Season with half the salt and pepper and place it in the pan.
4. After cooking for 3 minutes, flip sides and cook the other side for 3 minutes.
5. Remove pork with a slotted spoon and place on a plate.
6. Add butter and Dijon mustard into the same pan and keep stirring. When butter melts, add flour and stock and constantly stir until slightly thick.
7. Stir in the rest of the salt and pepper and simmer for a minute. Scrape the bottom of the pan to dislodge any pork particles.
8. Pour sauce over the pork medallions and serve.

LAMB STEW

Serves: 6

Nutritional values per serving:

Calories – 330

Fat – 9.3 g

Total Carbohydrate – 26.8 g

Protein – 34.3 g

Ingredients:

- 1.3 pounds diced lamb
- 1 pound carrots
- 3.5 ounces leeks
- 1.3 pounds potatoes
- 1-ounce dry gravy granules
- 2 beef stock cubes
- Water, as required

Directions:

1. Place lamb, carrots, leeks, potatoes, beef stock cubes, and dry gravy granules into a casserole dish. Pour enough water to cover the mixture. Mix well.
2. Cover the dish and place the casserole dish in an oven that has been preheated to 400°F and bake until meat is cooked. It should take 2 – 3 hours.
3. You can also cook it in a crock-pot if you own one.

CREAMY CHERRY TOMATO & SUMMER SQUASH PASTA

Serves: 2

Nutritional values per serving:

Calories – 357

Fat – 17.7 g

Total Carbohydrate – 44.1 g

Protein – 9.6 g

Ingredients:

- 4 ounces rotini or fusilli or penne pasta
- 1 medium yellow squash, cut into quarters lengthwise first and cut each into ¼ inch pieces
- 1 tablespoon olive oil
- 1 tablespoon lemon juice
- ½ ounce goat cheese, crumbled
- Few fresh basil leaves, chopped, to garnish
- 1 cup whole cherry tomatoes

- 1/8 teaspoon red pepper flakes or to taste
- ½ medium zucchini, cut into quarters lengthwise and cut each into ¼ inch pieces
- Salt to taste
- 1 tablespoon butter or olive oil
- Freshly ground black pepper to taste
- 2 small cloves garlic, peeled, minced

Directions:

1. Prepare a rimmed baking sheet by lining it with parchment paper.
2. Place cherry tomatoes, squash, and zucchini on a baking sheet. Drizzle oil over it and toss well.
3. Spread the vegetables in a single layer. Season with salt and pepper.
4. Place the baking sheet in an oven that has been preheated to 400°F and bake until the vegetables are cooked. It should take around 25 to 30 minutes. Make sure to stir the vegetables halfway through baking and rearrange the vegetables in a single layer.
5. In the meantime, cook the pasta following the instructions on the package. Drain the pasta and retain about ½ – ¾ cup of the cooking water.
6. Add the drained pasta into the pot in which it was cooked. Add butter, garlic, lemon juice, goat cheese, and red pepper flakes and toss well.
7. Add the retained cooked water and toss lightly, until the pasta is well coated in the mixture.
8. Add the roasted vegetables, along with the cooked liquid, and toss lightly.

9. Add salt and pepper to taste.
10. Divide the pasta into 2 bowls. Garnish with basil and serve.

LEMON PEPPER SHRIMP SCAMPI

Serves: 2

Nutritional values per serving: ½ cup orzo mixture and 7 shrimp

Calories – 403

Fat – 10.4 g

Total Carbohydrate – 34.7 g

Protein – 40.1 g

Ingredients:

- ½ cup uncooked orzo
- ¼ teaspoon salt, divided
- ¾ pound jumbo shrimp, peeled, deveined
- 1 tablespoon fresh lemon juice
- 1 tablespoon chopped fresh parsley
- 3 ½ teaspoons unsalted butter, divided
- 1 teaspoon minced, fresh garlic
- 1/8 teaspoon freshly ground pepper

Directions:

1. Follow the instructions on the package and cook orzo but do not add salt and fat while cooking.
2. Add the drained orzo into a bowl along with parsley and half the salt. Toss well and cover the bowl. Set it aside.
3. Meanwhile, place a nonstick skillet over medium-high flame. Add ½ tablespoon butter and let it melt.
4. Season shrimp with remaining salt and add into the pan. Cook shrimp for 2 minutes or until nearly cooked.
5. Remove shrimp onto a plate.
6. Add the rest of the butter into the pan. Once butter melts, add garlic and keep stirring for about ½ a minute.
7. Add shrimp back into the pan. Add lemon juice and pepper as well. Mix well. Cook until shrimp is fully cooked.
8. Serve hot with orzo.

SALMON WITH CREAMY DILL SAUCE

Serves: 3

Nutritional values per serving: 1 fillet with 2 tablespoons dill sauce

Calories – 418

Fat – 33 g

Total Carbohydrate – 3 g

Protein – 26 g

Ingredients:

- 3 salmon fillets (4 ounces each)
- ½ teaspoon onion salt
- 3 lemon slices
- ½ – ¾ teaspoon lemon-pepper seasoning
- ½ small onion, cut into rounds and separate the rings
- 1/8 cup cubed butter

For Dill Sauce:

- 3 tablespoons sour cream
- ½ tablespoon finely chopped onion
- ½ teaspoon prepared horseradish
- 1/8 teaspoon garlic salt
- 3 tablespoons mayonnaise
- ½ teaspoon lemon juice
- ½ teaspoon dried dill
- Pepper to taste

Directions:

1. Prepare a baking dish by lining it with a large sheet of heavy-duty foil hanging over the edges of the dish. Spray cooking spray over it.
2. Place the fillets in the pan, with the skin side facing down. Season with onion salt and lemon-pepper seasoning.
3. Place onion rings on top along with a slice of lemon on each fillet. Scatter butter cubes on top of the fillets.
4. Wrap the salmon with the extra foil that is hanging over.
5. Place the baking dish in an oven that has been preheated to 350°F and bake for 20 minutes.
6. Set the oven to broil mode. Uncover and broil for 4 to 6 minutes.
7. To make dill sauce: Add all the ingredients for dill sauce into a bowl and whisk well.
8. Serve fillets with dill sauce.

CREAMY CHICKEN & MUSHROOMS

Serves: 2

Nutritional values per serving: 1 cutlet with ¼ cup sauce

Calories – 324.8

Fat – 19.6 g

Total Carbohydrate – 4.2 g

Protein – 29.1 g

Ingredients:

- 2 chicken cutlets (5 ounces each)
- ¼ cup dry white wine
- 1 tablespoon finely chopped parsley
- ¼ teaspoon salt
- 2 cups mixed mushrooms, sliced if desired
- ¼ cup heavy cream
- ¼ teaspoon pepper
- 1 tablespoon canola oil

Directions:

1. Season chicken cutlets with 1/8-teaspoon salt and 1/8 teaspoon pepper.
2. Place a skillet over medium flame. Add half the oil and let it heat. Once the oil is heated, add chicken and cook until brown all over and cooked inside. It should take 8 – 10 minutes.
3. Remove chicken with a slotted spoon and place on a plate.
4. Add remaining oil into the skillet. Add mushrooms and cook until brown.
5. Raise the heat to high heat and pour wine. Let it boil until nearly dry.
6. Lower the heat and add cream, 1/8-teaspoon salt, and 1/8-teaspoon pepper.
7. Add chicken with the cooked juices and mix well.
8. Garnish with parsley and serve.

FETTUCCINE ALFREDO WITH CHICKEN AND BROCCOLI

Serves: 3

Nutritional values per serving:

Calories – 320

Fat – 8 g

Total Carbohydrate – 35 g

Protein – 27 g

Ingredients:

- 4 ounces fettuccine or linguine
- 1 tablespoon all-purpose flour
- ¼ cup grated Parmesan cheese
- A pinch of grated nutmeg or more to suit your taste
- 6 ounces broccoli, fresh or frozen, cut into bite-size florets
- ½ tablespoon butter
- Pepper to taste
- ¾ cup low-fat buttermilk

- 1/8 teaspoon dried thyme
- ½ pound grilled chicken breast, cut into bite-size pieces
- ¼ teaspoon salt

Directions:

1. Cook pasta following the instructions on the package. Drain and set aside.
2. Place a deep skillet over medium flame. Add butter. When butter melts, add flour and constantly stir for about a minute.
3. Add buttermilk, stirring constantly.
4. When it begins to boil, lower the heat and add Parmesan, nutmeg, and thyme. Stir until cheese melts.
5. Add broccoli and chicken and mix well. Cook until broccoli turns bright green.
6. Add salt and pepper to taste. Add pasta and stir until well coated.
7. Serve hot.

SWISS STEAK WITH CREAMY MASHED CAULIFLOWER

Serves: 3

Calories – 262.4

Fat – 12.2 g

Total Carbohydrate – 7.2 g

Protein – 28.6 g

Ingredients:

For Swiss Steak:

- 2 tablespoons all-purpose flour
- ¼ teaspoon black pepper
- 1 tablespoon vegetable oil
- ½ can (from a 14.5 ounces can) diced tomatoes
- ½ teaspoon onion powder
- ½ teaspoon salt
- 1 pound beef round steak, 1 inch thick
- 2 – 3 tablespoons water or more if required
- ¼ cup minced green bell pepper

For Creamy Mashed Cauliflower:

- 1.1 pounds cauliflower florets
- 1 tablespoon unsalted butter
- 2 tablespoons sour cream
- Salt to taste
- 1 clove garlic, peeled
- 2 tablespoons shredded Parmesan cheese
- ½ – 1 ½ tablespoons water
- Pepper to taste

To Garnish Creamy Mashed Cauliflower:

- Melted butter
- Pepper
- 1 tablespoon chopped parsley

Directions:

1. To make Swiss steak: Spread a sheet of parchment paper on your countertop. Place meat over it.
2. Combine flour, 1/8-teaspoon black pepper, and ¼ teaspoon salt in a bowl.
3. Sprinkle this mixture over the meat. Beat the steak with a meat mallet so that the flour mixture adheres to the steak.
4. Place a skillet over medium flame. Add oil and let it heat. Place beef in the pan and cook until the underside is golden brown. Turn the steak over and cook the other side until golden brown.
5. Lower the heat and add water into the skillet. Mix well and cook covered until meat is cooked through.

6. Sprinkle more water whenever required so that it doesn't burn.
7. Meanwhile, add tomatoes, onion powder, bell pepper, remaining pepper, and salt into a bowl and toss well.
8. Add this mixture into the skillet and mix well. Stir occasionally until the sauce is thick.
9. To make mashed cauliflower: Add water into a pot (half fill the pot). Place the pot over a high flame. When it begins to boil, drop the garlic and cauliflower florets into the pot and cook until absolutely soft.
10. Drain the cauliflower, retaining about a cup of the cooked water.
11. Add drained cauliflower into the food processor bowl. Add sour cream, cheese, and pepper and blend until smooth.
12. Add cooked water, a little at a time, if required (if you find the mash too thick, add water to get the consistency you desire).
13. Pour cauliflower puree into a serving bowl. Drizzle melted butter on top.
14. Garnish with pepper and parsley.
15. Serve Swiss steak with creamy cauliflower mash.

CREAMY PORK WITH SOUR CREAM SAUCE

Serves: 4

Nutritional values per serving:

Calories – 685.1

Fat – 52.9 g

Total Carbohydrate – 15.8 g

Protein – 35.7 g

Ingredients:

- 1 small egg, lightly beaten
- ¼ teaspoon crushed, dried rosemary
- 1/8 teaspoon garlic powder
- 1 ½ pounds pork steak cubes
- 1 tablespoon butter
- ½ can (from a 10.5 ounces can) condensed cream of chicken soup
- ¼ cup chicken broth

- ½ tablespoon water
- 1/8 teaspoon ground black pepper
- 1 ½ tablespoons vegetable oil
- ½ cup seasoned breadcrumbs
- 6 ounces fresh mushrooms, chopped
- ½ cup sour cream

Directions:

1. Spray a baking dish with cooking spray.
2. Add egg, rosemary, garlic powder, pepper, and water into a bowl and whisk well.
3. Place breadcrumbs in a shallow bowl.
4. Place a skillet over medium flame. Add oil and let it heat.
5. Meanwhile, dip the pork cubes in the egg mixture, one at a time.
6. Shaking off excess egg, dredge the meat pieces in breadcrumbs and place on a plate.
7. Once you are done with breading the pork cubes, place the breaded pork in the pan. Cook until brown all over.
8. Remove pork with a slotted spoon and place in a baking dish.
9. Add butter into the skillet. Once butter melts, add mushrooms and cook until slightly brown.
10. Add condensed cream of chicken soup, broth, and sour cream and stir until well combined. Heat thoroughly. Turn off the heat.
11. Pour the soup mixture all over the pork in the baking dish. Keep the dish covered with aluminum foil.

12. Place the casserole dish in an oven that has been preheated to 350°F and bake for about 40 – 45 minutes or until meat is well cooked inside.

QUICK ROAST CHICKEN & ROOT VEGETABLES

Serves: 2

Nutritional values per serving:

Calories – 332.5

Fat – 10.4 g

Total Carbohydrate – 28.6 g

Protein – 30.8 g

Ingredients:

- ½ pound turnips, peeled, cut into ½ inch chunks
- 1 tablespoons extra-virgin olive oil, divided
- Salt to taste
- 2 tablespoons all-purpose flour
- 1 bone-in chicken breasts, skinless, trimmed of fat, halved crosswise
- ½ pound baby potatoes, quartered
- ½ tablespoon chopped fresh marjoram or ½ teaspoon dried marjoram

- ¼ teaspoon freshly ground pepper
- ½ cup low-sodium chicken broth
- ½ large shallot, chopped
- 1 teaspoon red or white wine vinegar
- ½ tablespoon Dijon mustard

Directions:

1. Place potatoes and turnips in a bowl. Drizzle ½ tablespoon oil. Sprinkle about ¼ teaspoon salt, marjoram, and 1/8 teaspoon pepper and toss well.
2. Transfer the vegetables onto a baking sheet and spread it evenly.
3. Place the baking sheet in an oven that has been preheated to 500°F and roast for 15 minutes. Turn the vegetables halfway through roasting.
4. In the meantime, whisk together 1-teaspoon flour and broth in a bowl.
5. Sprinkle 1/8-teaspoon salt and 1/8 teaspoon pepper over the chicken.
6. Place remaining flour on a plate. Coat the chicken pieces in flour. Shake off extra flour from the chicken.
7. Place a large skillet over medium flame. Add ½ tablespoon of oil and let it heat.
8. Once the oil is heated, place chicken in the pan cook until the underside is golden brown.
9. Flip sides and cook the other side until golden brown.
10. Remove the chicken from the pan using a slotted spoon and place it on the baking sheet along with vegetables.

11. Continue baking until chicken is well cooked inside.
12. Place the skillet back over heat (during the last 10 minutes of baking). Add shallots and sauté for a couple of minutes.
13. Add the broth – flour mixture and constantly stir until it comes to a boil.
14. Lower the heat and simmer until half its original quantity.
15. Add mustard and vinegar and mix well. Turn off the heat.
16. Divide chicken and vegetables onto 2 serving plates. Serve with sauce.

ROSEMARY-LEMON LAMB CHOPS WITH POTATO AND FENNEL LATKES

Serves: 2

Nutritional values per serving: 2 lamb chops with latkes

Calories – 276

Fat – 12 g

Total Carbohydrate – 19 g

Protein – 23 g

Ingredients:

- 1 medium russet potatoes, peeled, shredded
- 2 tablespoons finely chopped onion
- 2 cloves garlic, minced
- 4 lamb rib chops (3 ounces each), 1 inch thick, trimmed of fat
- 1 small egg white
- Pepper to taste
- ½ medium fennel bulb, peeled, cored, shredded

- ½ tablespoon chopped fresh rosemary
- ½ teaspoon finely shredded lemon zest
- ½ tablespoon canola oil
- Salt to taste

Directions:

1. To make latkes: Add potato, onion, and fennel into a microwave-safe bowl. Cover the bowl with plastic wrap.
2. Make a couple of holes on the wrap and cook on high in a microwave until vegetables are slightly soft.
3. Stir after every minute while cooking. Let the mixture cool to room temperature. Squeeze the vegetables of excess moisture.
4. In the meantime, add rosemary, lemon zest, a pinch of salt and pepper into a bowl and mix well. Scatter this mixture over the lamb. Rub it well into it.
5. Place a grill pan over medium flame. Spray the pan with cooking spray. When pan heats, place the lamb chops and cook until the way you prefer it cooked; 12 – 14 minutes for medium-rare and 15 – 17 minutes for rare.
6. Add egg white into the bowl of potato – fennel – onion mixture along with salt and pepper to taste. Mix well.
7. Make 4 equal portions of the mixture.
8. Place a nonstick pan over medium-high flame. Add oil and let it heat.
9. Place the latkes in the pan and flatten into a round shape, ½ inch thick.

10. Cook until the underside is golden brown. Turn the latkes over and cook the other side until golden brown.
11. Serve lamb chops with latkes.

EASY PAELLA

Serves: 4

Nutritional values per serving:

Calories – 736.2

Fat – 35.1 g

Total Carbohydrate – 45.7 g

Protein – 55.7 g

Ingredients:

- 3 tablespoons olive oil, divided
- 1 teaspoon dried oregano
- 1 pound skinless, boneless chicken breasts, cut into 2-inch pieces
- 2 cloves garlic, crushed
- 1 cup uncooked, short-grain white rice, rinsed
- 2 small bay leaves
- 2 cups chicken stock
- ½ Spanish onion, chopped

- ½ pound chorizo sausage, discard casings, crumbled
- ½ tablespoon paprika
- Salt to taste
- ½ teaspoon crushed red pepper flakes
- 8 – 10 threads saffron
- A handful fresh Italian flat-leaf parsley, chopped
- Zest of a lemon, grated
- ½ red bell pepper, chopped
- ½ pound shrimp, peeled, deveined

Directions:

1. Add 1-tablespoon oil, oregano, pepper, paprika, and salt into a bowl and mix well.
2. Add chicken and mix until chicken is well coated with the mixture.
3. Keep the bowl covered and chill for a couple of hours.
4. Place a large skillet over medium flame. Add 1 tablespoon of oil. When the oil is heated, add garlic, rice, and red pepper flakes and keep stirring for a couple of minutes, until rice is well coated with oil.
5. Add bay leaves, saffron threads, chicken stock, parsley, and lemon zest.
6. When it comes to a boil, lower the heat to medium-low. Cook for about 15 minutes.
7. In the meantime, place a skillet over medium flame. Add a tablespoon of oil. When the oil is heated, add onion and chicken and cook for 3 – 4 minutes.
8. Add bell pepper and crumbled sausage and mix well. Stir often for 3 – 4 minutes.

9. Add shrimp and stir. Cook until shrimp turns pink. Flip sides of the shrimp and cook the other side until pink.
10. Take a large serving platter. Place the rice mixture over it and spread it evenly.
11. Place meat mixture on top and serve.

LAMB & RICE

Serves: 3

Nutritional values per serving: 2/3-cup lamb mixture with 1/3-cup rice

Calories – 330

Fat – 12 g

Total Carbohydrate – 21 g

Protein – 32 g

Ingredients:

- 1 pound boneless lamb shoulder, trimmed of fat, cut into bite-size cubes
- ¼ cup chopped onion
- ½ Serrano chili pepper, deseeded
- 3 cloves garlic, peeled, minced
- ½ teaspoon ground ginger
- ¼ teaspoon dry mustard
- A pinch of cayenne pepper

- ¼ cup snipped fresh cilantro
- ½ can (from a 14.5 ounces can) diced tomatoes with its liquid
- ½ teaspoon ground coriander
- 1/8 teaspoon salt
- 1 cup hot, cooked brown rice

Directions:

1. Add tomatoes, garlic, ginger, onion, chili pepper, mustard, cayenne pepper, coriander, and salt into a bowl and mix well.
2. Place lamb in a Dutch oven. Place the pot over a low flame.
3. Add the tomato mixture over the lamb and mix well. Cover and cook until meat is tender. You can also cook it in a slow cooker if you own one.
4. Divide rice onto 3 plates. Remove lamb with a slotted spoon and divide among the plates (place it over the rice).
5. Remove fat that is floating on top (from the Dutch oven). Pour the tomato mixture over the lamb.
6. Sprinkle cilantro on top and serve.

GRILLED FENNEL-CUMIN LAMB CHOPS

Serves: 4

Nutritional values per serving:

Calories – 239.4

Fat – 12.1 g

Total Carbohydrate – 1.6 g

Protein – 29.1 g

Ingredients:

- 8 lamb rib chops, 1 inch thick, trimmed of fat
- 1 ½ teaspoons fennel seeds, crushed
- ½ teaspoon salt
- ¼ teaspoon ground black pepper
- 2 large cloves garlic, peeled, minced
- 1 ½ teaspoons ground cumin
- ½ teaspoon ground coriander

Directions:

1. Add garlic, cumin, coriander, fennel seeds, coriander, and black pepper into a small bowl and stir well. Sprinkle this mixture over the chops. Rub it well into it.
2. Place chops on a plate. Cover the meat with cling wrap and chill for 1 – 24 hours.
3. Remove the meat from the refrigerator 30 minutes before grilling.
4. Set up your grill and preheat to medium heat.
5. Place the chops on the rack and cook for 10 – 14 minutes for medium-rare and 14 – 16 minutes for medium.
6. Serve hot.

STRAWBERRY ICE CREAM

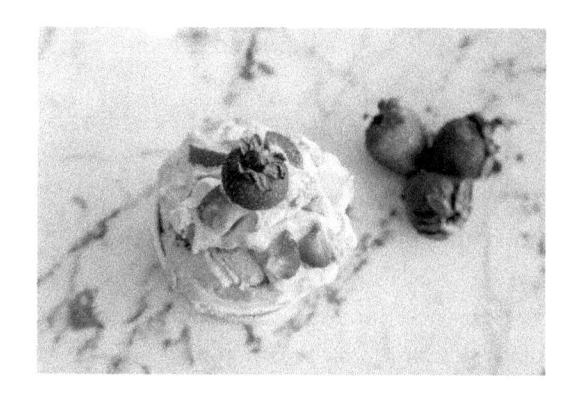

Serves: 4

Nutritional values per serving:

Calories – 354.2

Fat – 23.4 g

Total Carbohydrate – 34.1 g

Protein – 3.6 g

Ingredients:

- 1 cup whole milk
- ½ cup white sugar
- 1 teaspoon vanilla extract
- 1 drop red food coloring
- 1 cup heavy cream
- 1/8 teaspoon salt
- 1 cup mashed, fresh strawberries

Directions:

1. Add milk, sugar, vanilla, food coloring, cream, salt, and strawberries into a bowl and stir until sugar dissolves completely.
2. Cover the bowl and place it in the freezer for 30 minutes.
3. Set up your ice cream maker. Follow the manufacturer's instructions and churn the ice cream.
4. Serve right away for a soft-serve consistency.
5. If you prefer harder ice cream, transfer the mixture into a freezer-safe container. Freeze until firm.

PEACH COBBLER

Serves: 18

Nutritional values per serving: Without serving options

Calories – 386

Fat – 12 g

Total Carbohydrate – 66 g

Protein – 4 g

Ingredients:

- 10 peaches, peeled, sliced (8 cups)
- ½ teaspoon salt
- 1 ½ cups granulated sugar
- For batter:
- ¾ cup butter, chilled
- 2 cups granulated sugar
- ½ teaspoon salt
- 2 teaspoons ground cinnamon

- 2 cups all-purpose flour
- 4 teaspoons baking powder
- 1 ½ cups milk

Serving Options: Use Any

- Vanilla ice cream
- Heavy cream
- Whipping cream

Directions:

1. Place a saucepan over medium flame. Add peaches, salt, and sugar and mix well. Stir occasionally. When sugar dissolves, turn off the heat.
2. Cut the chilled butter into slices and place the butter slices in a large baking dish (13 x 9 inches).
3. Place the baking dish in the oven and set the oven to 350°F. Switch on the oven and let the butter melt.
4. As soon as the butter melts, take out the baking dish from the oven.
5. Add flour, baking powder, sugar, and salt into a large bowl and stir until well incorporated.
6. Add milk and stir until just incorporated, making sure not to over-mix.
7. Spoon the mixture into the pan, over the melted butter. Make sure that the batter is spread smoothly and evenly.
8. Dust with cinnamon. Be generous and use more if required.
9. Place the baking dish back in the oven and bake for about 40 – 50 minutes.

10. Remove the baking dish from the oven and let it cool until it is warm.
11. Serve with any one of the serving options.

CRANBERRY & RUBY GRAPEFRUIT COMPOTE

Serves: 12

Nutritional values per serving: ¾ cup

Calories – 140

Fat – 0 g

Total Carbohydrate – 36 g

Protein – 1 g

Ingredients:

- 3 ½ cups fresh or frozen cranberries
- 4-5 thin strips orange zest
- ¼ cup sugar
- 1 ½ large red grapefruit, peel, deseeded, separate segments, discard membrane
- 10 tablespoons water
- 1-inch cinnamon stick (optional)
- ¼ cup orange juice
- Fresh mint sprigs to garnish

Directions:

1. Add cranberries, orange zest, sugar, water, cinnamon stick, and orange juice to a saucepan. Stir well.
2. Place the saucepan over medium-high heat. Cook until the cranberries are tender, stirring occasionally. When you see that the cranberries have started popping, turn off the heat.
3. Spoon the cranberries into a bowl and chill for at least 2 hours after the cranberries have cooled completely.
4. Remove the bowl from the refrigerator. Add the grapefruits to it. Mix well.
5. Serve in individual bowls, garnished with mint sprigs. Refrigerate until use. It can last for 2 days if refrigerated.
6. When this compote is served for breakfast, serve it with plain yogurt. When you serve it for dessert, serve it with frozen vanilla yogurt.

CONCLUSION

The chaos and stress of the modern lifestyle are the primary reason for the various health problems that currently plague humanity. To lead a healthy life, you need to concentrate on your diet, exercise, and sleep. A healthy diet directly influences your physical and mental wellbeing. If the diet is devoid of essential nutrients or increases the intake of unhealthy foods, your body cannot function optimally. Therefore, the first step toward regaining control of your health is to concentrate on your diet.

The low-oxalate diet is a simple yet effective meal plan that helps tackle and reverse several health problems associated with oxalate stone formation. There is a lot to gain from tackling irritable bowel syndrome to kidney stones and restoring your energy levels while reducing chronic fatigue. As promised, this book is filled with helpful information and practical tips you can use to restore your overall health.

In this book, you were introduced to the concept of oxalates and how your body processes them. By learning about oxalates and oxalate stone formation, you get a better

Conclusion

understanding of the role nutrition plays in your health. The comprehensive low-oxalate diet food list provided makes it incredibly simple to follow this diet. The practical and actionable tips discussed will help you attain its many benefits.

This book also includes several diet recipes that are not only easy to understand but simple to cook too. You can enjoy a healthy, wholesome, and delicious low-oxalate diet home-cooked meal within no time. Forget about spending hours together in the kitchen to cook meals! These recipes will not only improve your health, they will strengthen your relationship with food. Stock your pantry with low-oxalate diet ingredients, select a recipe that strikes your fancy, and follow the instructions. That's about it!

So, what are you waiting for? Now that you are armed with all the information about the low-oxalate diet, it is time to implement the simple tips and suggestions given in this book. There is no time like the present to get started because the key to good health lies in your hands! While transitioning to this new diet, don't forget to be patient with yourself.

Strictly follow this diet, and see the positive change in your overall health and wellbeing.